better nutrition *magazine* presents

WEIGHT LOSS

by KATE RHÉAUME-BLEUE, ND

better nutrition healthy living guide

Acknowledgements

I would like to thank Dr. Michael Lyon and Dr. Michael Murray, and Atria Press, publishers of *Hunger Free Forever* for all the data and science behind the Hunger Free Forever Weight Management Program.

Published by:
Active Interest Media, Inc.
300 N. Continental Blvd., Suite 650
El Segundo, CA 90245

This booklet is part of the *Better Nutrition Healthy Living Guide* series. For more information, visit www.betternutrition.com. Better Nutrition magazine is available at fine natural health stores throughout the United States. Design by Aline Design: Bellingham, Wash.

WEIGHT LOSS

CONTENTS

better nutrition healthy living guide

Introduction

Why Diets Don't Work

Millions of people have learned the hard way that diets don't work. Statistics from the National Institutes of Health tell us that 98 percent of people who lose weight by "going on a diet" end up gaining it back within five years—and 90 percent of those people gain back more weight than they lost.

Diets can increase your appetite as you lose weight, making it harder to resist temptation. They can also cause muscle loss, which lowers metabolic rate, turning more of your extra calories into fat. Plus, restrictive diets don't help you make changes you can live with for very long, so you tend to give up or give in.

People continue to diet, even though their odds of success are slim. We all know that the recipe for success at weight loss is "eat less and exercise more," but that is easier said than done. In fact, eating less and exercising more is almost impossible for the average overweight person when their appetite is out of control. With the body sending out powerful signals saying "EAT," how do you change bad habits to lose weight sensibly? What if you could turn the hunger switch off? Then you might be able to gain control of your appetite and achieve your weight loss goals.

According to Drs. Michael Lyon and Michael Murray in their book, *Hunger Free Forever*, the key to effective and lasting weight loss is not dieting or deprivation. Instead, permanent weight loss comes from eliminating excessive hunger and increasing the pleasure and satisfaction you get from food. Major discoveries in the field of appetite control have uncovered the answer to safe and effective lifelong weight control.

The Size of The Problem

Over the past 50 years, changes in food technology, transportation and agriculture have created an unprecedented increase in the availability of food throughout most of the world. This seems to have led to an obesity epidemic. According to the World Health Organization, out of the world's six billion people, one billion are overweight compared to 800 million who are undernourished. America has the world's highest percentage of obese people, as well as the highest number of people succumbing to obesity-related illnesses.

The simplest definition of obesity is an excessive amount of body fat. Being overweight is not the same as being fat. Being overweight simply means an excess of body weight relative to height. For example, a muscular athlete may be heavy, yet have a low percentage of body fat.

The body mass index (BMI) is now the accepted standard for classifying body composition. The BMI is found by dividing a person's weight in kilograms by their height in meters squared. Unless you are a fan of the metric system or like math problems, you can use the simple table below. Find your height (in inches) in the left-hand column. Look across the row to your weight. The number at the top of that column is your BMI.

Table 1.1 **Body Mass Index (BMI) Chart**

BMI (kg/m^2)	19	20	21	22	23	24	25	26	27	28	29	30	35	40
Height (in.)	Weight (lb.)													
58	91	96	100	105	110	115	119	124	129	134	138	143	167	191
59	94	99	104	109	114	119	124	128	133	138	143	148	173	198
60	97	102	107	112	118	123	128	133	138	143	148	153	179	204
61	100	106	111	116	122	127	132	137	143	148	153	158	185	211
62	104	109	115	120	126	131	136	142	147	153	158	164	191	218
63	107	113	118	124	130	135	141	146	152	158	163	169	197	225
64	110	116	122	128	134	140	145	151	157	163	169	174	204	232
65	114	120	126	132	138	144	150	156	162	168	174	180	210	240
66	118	124	130	136	142	148	155	161	167	173	179	186	216	247
67	121	127	134	140	146	153	159	166	172	178	185	191	223	255
68	125	131	138	144	151	158	164	171	177	184	190	197	230	262
69	128	135	142	149	155	162	169	176	182	189	196	203	236	270
70	132	139	146	153	160	167	174	181	188	195	202	207	243	278
71	136	143	150	157	165	172	179	186	193	200	208	215	250	286
72	140	147	154	162	169	177	184	191	199	206	213	221	258	294
73	144	151	159	166	174	182	189	197	204	212	219	227	265	302
74	148	155	163	171	179	186	194	202	210	218	225	233	272	311
75	152	160	168	176	184	192	200	208	216	224	232	240	279	319
76	156	164	172	180	189	197	205	213	221	230	238	246	287	328

A BMI between 25 and 29 suggests you are overweight, while a BMI of 30 or greater indicates obesity. A BMI of 40 or greater is referred to as morbid obesity and is associated with extreme health risks.

Your waist circumference combined with your BMI can be a very good indicator of your risk for the diseases associated with obesity, especially the major killers like heart disease, stroke, cancer and diabetes.

Table 1.2 **Risk of Associated Disease According to BMI And Waist Size**

BMI		Waist less than or equal to 40 in. (men) or 35 in. (women)	Waist greater than 40 in. (men) or 35 in. (women)
18.5 or less	Underweight	--	N/A
18.5 - 24.9	Normal	--	N/A
25.0 - 29.9	Overweight	Increased	High
30.0 - 34.9	Obese	High	Very High
35.0 - 39.9	Obese	Very High	Very High
40 or greater	Extremely Obese	Extremely High	Extremely High

Approximately 65 million American adults are now obese—more than the total populations of Britain, France or Italy. As alarming as these statistics are, it is perhaps more alarming that there is no end in sight. Obesity is now regarded as the major cause of death in the United States. Without question, American baby boomers and subsequent generations have been influenced by both food marketing and food technology in ways similar to the tactics used by tobacco companies that resulted in millions of people becoming addicted to cigarettes.

While other factors may be involved, obesity is caused primarily by eating more calories than are needed to operate your body. High calorie, low nutrient foods can taste good, but they don't satisfy a hungry body for long. With a full understanding of appetite and satiety, you can prevent obesity, Type 2 diabetes and related chronic diseases.

What is Satiety?

Satiety occurs when a person feels full or gratified to the point of satisfaction. Humans eat to achieve satiety. But people who are overweight have a resistance to satiety that makes them eat more. They are also likely to have frequent food cravings. Understanding this phenomenon can help you take control of your appetite—no matter what your weight loss goal is.

Unlike other "diets," this booklet focuses on reducing appetite and eliminating unhealthy food cravings. You can feel satisfied, even with significant reductions in the amount you eat. By retraining your appetite and metabolism, you can change your relationship with food and change your life!

Major Health Risks Associated with Obesity

Cardiovascular System
Chronic venous insufficiency, deep vein thrombosis, varicose veins
Hypertension
Hyperlipidemia (high cholesterol and triglycerides)
Atherosclerosis (hardening of the arteries)
Peripheral vascular disease

Digestive System
Gastroesophageal reflux disease (heartburn)
Gallbladder disease
Nonalcoholic steatohepatitis (fatty liver disease)

Reproductive System
Infertility
Menstrual abnormalities
Pregnancy abnormalities
Hirsutism (excessive hair growth in females)
Impotence
Polycystic ovary syndrome (PCOS)
Neural tube birth defects

Nervous System
Carpal tunnel syndrome
Stroke
Dementia
Depression

Endocrine System
Insulin resistance
Type 2 diabetes
Pancreatitis
Musculoskeletal System
Osteoarthritis
Rheumatoid arthritis
Vertebral disk herniation
Degenerative joint disease
Inguinal hernia
Low back pain

Respiratory System
Asthma
Obesity hypoventilation syndrome
Sleep apnea
Pulmonary hypertension

Urinary System
Urinary stress incontinence
Increased uric acid
Renal disease

Dermatology System (Skin)
Cellulitis (inflammation or infection of the connective tissue of the skin)
Fungal skin infections

Immune System
Cancers (breast, prostate and colon)
Poor healing of wounds and infection

Excerpt from Hunger Free Forever

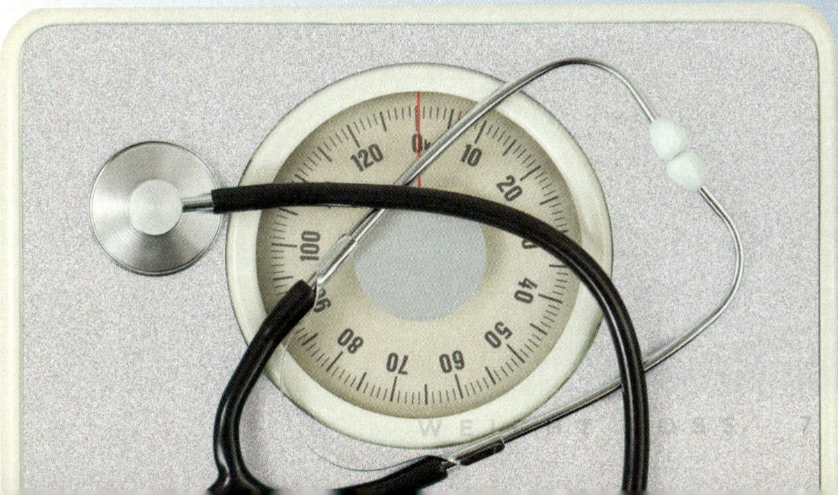

Chapter One

High Fiber Diet

Blood sugar and appetite are monitored by various systems within the body. For example, specialized immune cells that surround every brain cell can sense the level of glucose in your blood. Every time blood sugar drops rapidly, these cells send signals to parts of the brain that cause you to feel hungry. If you are overweight, insulin resistance and cravings can make your brain send out hunger signals even when it is inappropriate.

Fods high in soluble fiber—rolled oats, brown rice, apples

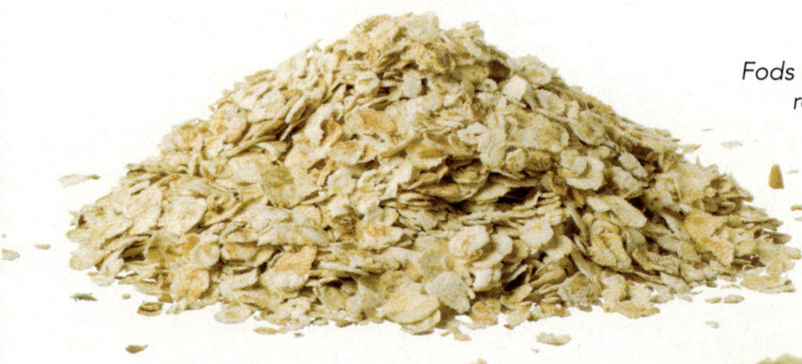

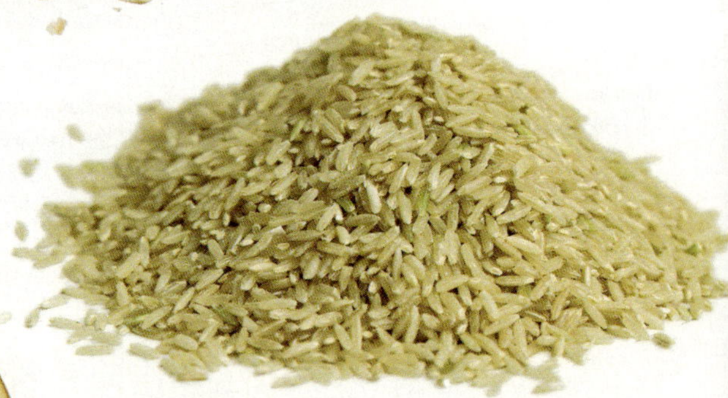

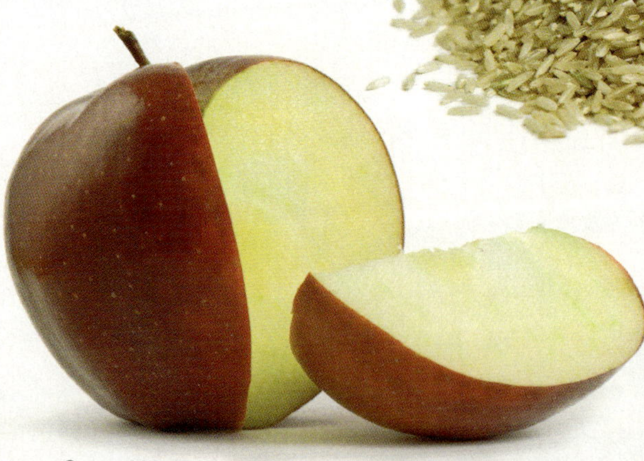

When your blood sugar levels routinely rise dramatically and then drop quickly (due to the secretion of insulin) you can develop insulin resistance. Your body doesn't respond as it should to insulin so more is needed and a vicious cycle develops. The "blood sugar roller coaster" is a good way to describe the phenomenon of blood glucose levels that rocket up and down. But this is one roller coaster you don't want to ride. These highs and lows are very hard on the body and can contribute to the dangerous complications of diabetes including blindness, nerve death and cardiovascular disease.

Importance of Soluble Fiber

A safe and effective route to weight loss is to greatly increase your consumption of dietary fiber. Unfortunately you would need very large amounts of ordinary fiber to achieve significant weight control—higher quantities than most people would be willing or able to eat. Doctors recommend you consume 30 grams of fiber per day, however most Americans eat a maximum of 15 grams of fiber daily. In reality, 75 to 100 grams per day of conventional dietary fiber would probably be required to produce a feeling of satiety in overweight individuals. But no one could eat that much regular fiber!

While bran and other non-soluble fibers support digestive health, it is soluble fiber that reduces appetite, balances blood sugar and lowers cholesterol. Soluble fibers are indigestible plant compounds that can absorb water. Their effectiveness at increasing satiety and improving blood sugar balance is directly proportionate to the amount of water the fiber can absorb and retain. The thickness or viscosity the fiber develops as it moves through the stomach and intestine is also a key to its effectiveness. For example, oat bran lowers cholesterol and controls blood sugar better than wheat bran because it absorbs more water.

Researchers have identified and isolated soluble dietary fibers that have extremely high viscosity and water holding capacity. These have been blended into a unique food ingredient and nutritional supplement called PGX® (short for PolyGlycoPlex®). The fibers in PGX multiply each other's effects, exerting health benefits that would be expected from much larger quantities of single fibers or other fiber blends.

PGX is an excellent example of how soluble fiber can enhance health. It has excellent gel-forming properties and absorbs hundreds of times its weight in water, creating volume and viscosity three to five times greater than single fibers like psyllium or oat bran. A 5 gram serving of PGX can produce the same volume and viscosity of fiber as four bowls of oat bran. This is a revolution in the science of satiety. Now small amounts of PGX can be consumed before meals and it will produce results equivalent to those previously only possible by eating enormous quantities of any other fiber!

PGX is the result of extensive university-based research resulting in this unique polysaccharide (fiber) complex. When added to food, this patent pending ingredient has been shown to reduce the glycemic index—a measure of how quickly and how much a particular food raises blood sugar.

According to Drs. Lyon and Murray, detailed clinical studies published in major medical journals and presented at major medical conferences have shown that PGX can:

- reduce appetite and promote effective weight loss;
- increase the body's levels of compounds that block appetite and promote satiety;
- decrease the levels of compounds that stimulate overeating;
- reduce postprandial (after-meal) blood glucose levels when added to or taken with foods;
- reduce the glycemic index of foods and beverages;
- promote healthy blood sugar control in the overweight and obese (already within normal range); and
- maintain healthy blood cholesterol and triglycerides (already within normal range).
- improve blood sugar control and increase the natural release of satiety-inducing hormones (already within the normal range); and
- help develop a life long healthy relationship with food.

It's important to note that PGX is not intended to treat, cure, or prevent any disease. It is a dietary supplement designed to support healthy weight loss.

Statistics indicate that, with the addition of sufficient soluble fiber to their diets, many people can lose between one to two-and-a-half pounds per week. Keep in mind, it is not recommended that you lose weight too rapidly as you can lose muscle mass as well. Gradual weight loss, combined with exercise to build muscle mass is the ideal, long-term solution to weight management.

Chapter Two

Blood Sugar And Appetite Control

In the *Hunger Free Forever* book, Dr. Murray and Dr. Lyon explain that gaining weight is like inviting a monster to live in your body. The monster is most at home when you have an accumulation of fat in the abdominal cavity and surrounding internal organs. This type of fat leads to insulin resistance and lifelong obesity. The monster's hunger is largely the result of action by two opposing hormones secreted by fat cells in the abdomen. Your body's levels of these fat-derived hormones influence your sensitivity to insulin. As you gain weight, your appetite and food cravings increase while your ability to feel satisfied by food decreases. It takes a lot to feed the monster.

Taming The Monster

Handling the appetite monster requires that you re-establish your body's sensitivity to insulin. When insulin sensitivity is restored, more nutrients enter muscle cells after each meal, making fewer calories available to fat cells and more calories available for energy and heat.

Incorporating highly soluble fiber into your daily diet helps reestablish a healthy balance between these hormones to help improve insulin sensitivity. Improving the body's sensitivity to insulin is absolutely key to controlling appetite, cravings and weight gain. Stabilizing blood sugar levels eliminates the roller coaster and most people find this makes it much easier to lose pounds. Of course you also need to identify and eliminate the bad habits that are sabotaging your weight loss efforts. With your appetite under control, a healthy lifestyle is easier to adopt and can help make your healthy weight a permanent way of life rather than the results of a constant effort to "diet."

Five Weight Loss Strategies That Work

- Restore blood sugar stability.
- Eat for high satiety.
- Rev up your metabolism.
- Reduce the effects of stress and cortisol.
- Tone your muscles, train your heart.

Resetting Your Appetite

Putting on weight when food was abundant was good survival strategy during prehistoric times since famine could be just around the corner. But today, we have a plentiful food supply. Yet, despite this abundancy, you will find it hard to adjust your eating behavior if your body is stuck in a "fat storing" mode .

A key to losing weight and keeping it off is keeping blood glucose (blood sugar) levels within a very narrow range. Landmark research has demonstrated that frequent and rapid swings in blood sugar magnify appetite and cause food cravings in individuals struggling with their weight. This blood sugar roller coaster is technically called glycemic volatility and it can be observed in most overweight people.

Research has shown that moderate dietary changes, with the addition of PGX, can eliminate glycemic volatility and promote overall good health. This improves the action of insulin, a key to achieving long-term weight goals. When blood sugar levels are stable, appetite and cravings are reduced.

Insulin And Blood Sugar Control

Dr. Murray explains it this way, "Think of insulin as a key that opens a cell's 'door' and lets in glucose—the basic food cells need. Around the clock, the pancreas secretes a small amount of insulin so some glucose can enter cells, keeping them alive and energized. After a meal, as the bloodstream becomes flooded with glucose, a surge of insulin is released from the pancreas. This causes sugar to be quickly transferred from the blood to organs, energizing them and keeping blood sugar levels from rising too high. But, when you start gaining weight, particularly belly fat, substances are also secreted from this fat tissue that promote insulin resistance. Insulin is released but it no longer works as effectively as it should. The insulin doesn't change, but the cells throughout the body lose some of their ability to recognize insulin and respond to it as they should."

If blood sugar levels drop too low, you die. If blood sugar levels go too high, you die. Low blood sugar is fairly easy to understand: Glucose is fuel for your body and if you run out of glucose, your body will quit. Most tissues get their energy from fat but the brain depends on glucose. In fact, if your blood glucose levels drop too low you can die in a few seconds. For this reason the body has sophisticated feedback and control mechanisms to ensure the brain receives a steady supply of glucose.

But when blood glucose levels are elevated, the excess glucose may bind itself to various body proteins and other molecules, changing their structure. The accumulation of these "sugar coated molecules" is a recognized factor in accelerated aging, and eventually death.

Because elevated blood sugar is very harmful, the body works hard to keep levels normal, in spite of insulin resistance. It does this by releasing higher amounts of insulin around the clock, particularly after meals. Under these conditions, if insulin levels did not rise substantially, diabetes would occur. The body fends off diabetes by secreting these high levels of insulin, but with serious implications for your health.

Here's the vicious cycle: When blood sugar surges after a meal, a massive release of insulin occurs. Even in the insulin resistant, cells eventually open up to glucose. The glucose surge is usually followed by a rapid drop in blood sugar. As blood sugar plummets, the brain, pancreas and liver sense the drop and declare an emergency. The brain is alarmed by any rapid drop in blood sugar and it does everything it can to get you to reach for a quick sugar

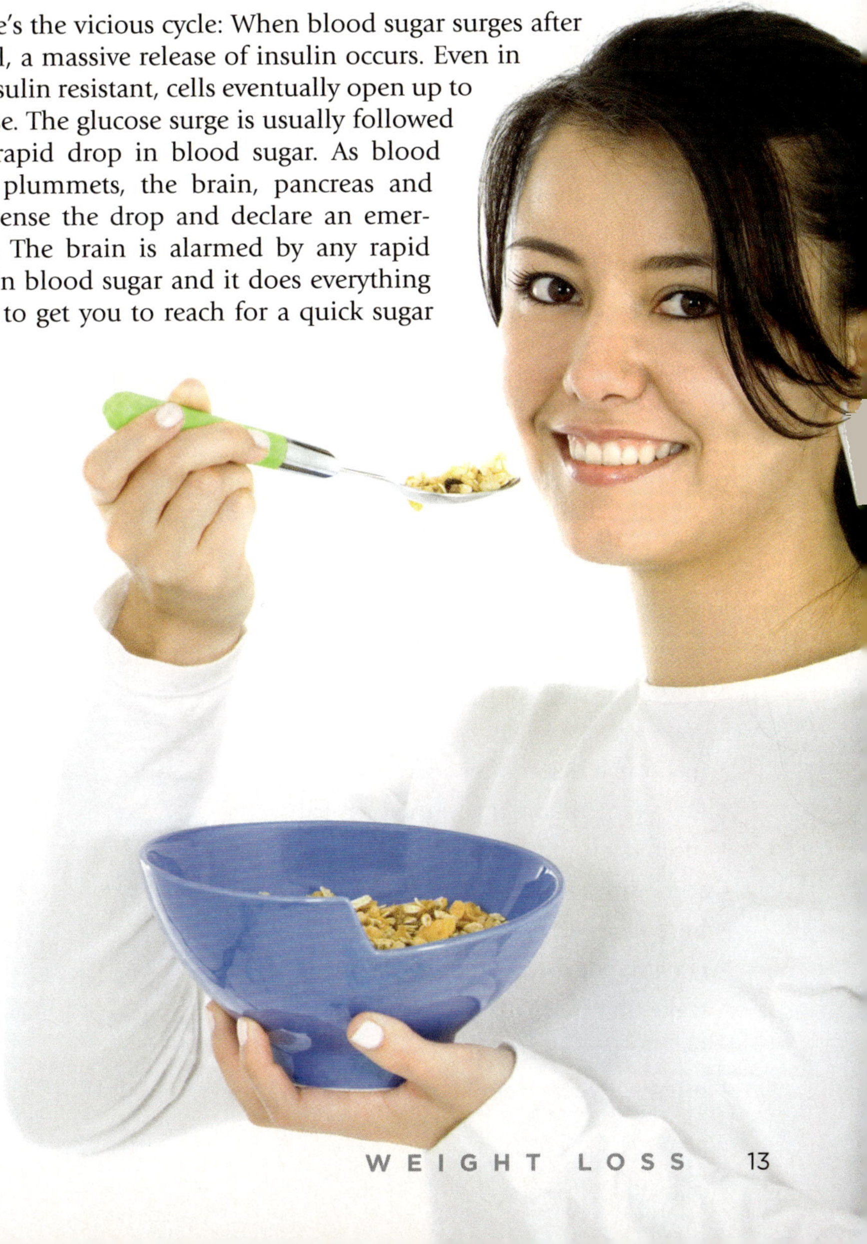

fix. To prevent severe low blood sugar (hypoglycemia), hormones such as glucagon, epinephrine (adrenalin) and cortisol are released. These promote the release of stored energy (glycogen) from the liver and muscles.

Blood Sugar Facts

- We get glucose from the carbohydrates we eat.
- High sugar, low fiber, starchy foods eaten in excess cause blood sugar levels to rise quickly.
- The body responds to an after-meal rise in blood glucose by secreting insulin.
- Insulin lowers blood glucose by increasing the rate at which glucose is taken up by cells throughout the body.
- Drops in blood glucose from fasting or exercise cause the release of glucagon, another hormone produced by the pancreas.
- Glucagon stimulates the release of glucose stored in the muscles and liver (glycogen).

If blood sugar levels fall sharply or if a person is angry or frightened, the hormones epinephrine (adrenalin) and corticosteroids (cortisol) may be released by the adrenal glands. These hormones provide quicker breakdown of stored glucose for extra energy during a crisis or increased need.

These mechanisms are designed to keep blood sugar levels within a very narrow range, but diet and lifestyle can unbalance the body's processes to cause obesity, diabetes and other blood sugar disorders.

Are You Riding The Blood Sugar Roller Coaster?

Do you . . .

- have a waist circumference larger than your hips?
- have difficulty losing weight?
- crave sweets?
- feel much better after you eat?
- feel very irritable if you miss a meal?
- often cry for no reason?
- sometimes feel "spacey" and distracted?
- have elevated blood sugar or triglyceride levels?
- get anxious for no apparent reason?
- wake up often during the night?
- feel hungry all the time?
- often get very sleepy in the afternoon?

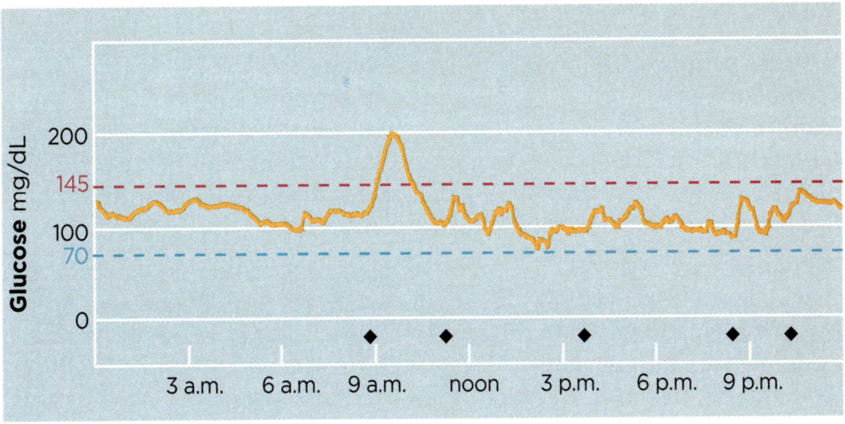

Figure 3.1 **Overweight adult before weight loss demonstrating elevated blood sugar (glycemic volatility)**

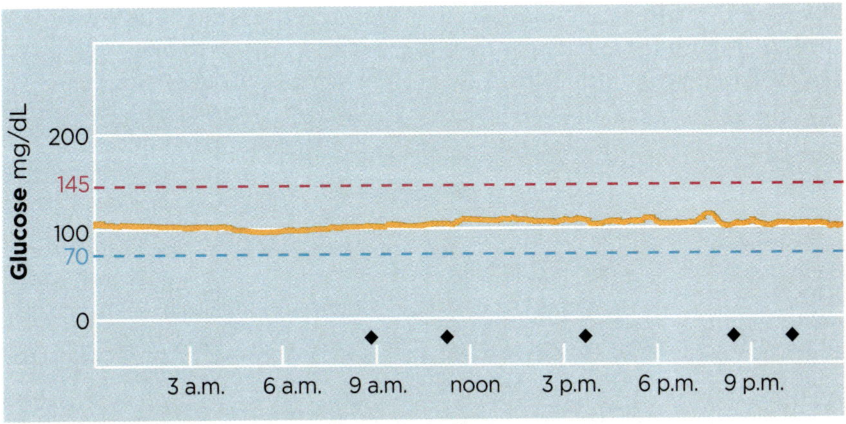

Figure 3.2 **Healthy 24 hour blood sugar graph of overweight adult after four weeks of using PGX.**

These symptoms are common in people with blood sugar volatility. Thanks to technology known as Continuous Glucose Monitoring (CGM) a tiny electronic device can measure blood sugar levels and send information every few seconds to a small, pager-sized computer module worn on the patient's belt. The blood sugar data can then be downloaded to a doctor's or researcher's computer. The graphs below are examples of average blood sugar readings taken every five minutes. Using this technology, doctors have discovered that people with weight problems often have highly fluctuating blood sugar which is directly related to their insulin resistance and a loss of blood sugar control.

Are You a Diabetic in Training?

Many people with insulin resistance develop Type 2 diabetes when their pancreas becomes too "tired" to keep producing massive amounts of insulin. People with insulin resistance will usually develop Type 2 diabetes before pancreatic production of insulin declines. This is the definition of Type 2 diabetes. When Type 2 diabetes is diagnosed, insulin levels are usually normal or elevated. Restoring insulin sensitivity is essential.

Pre-diabetes, also called "impaired glucose tolerance," is a condition that occurs when a person's blood glucose levels are higher than normal, but not high enough for a diagnosis of Type 2 diabetes. There are almost as many people in the United States with pre-diabetes (about 16 million) as there are diabetics. Although many of these people are told by their physicians that they just have "a touch of diabetes," research indicates that their insulin resistance is accompanied by serious health risks.

Anyone who is insulin resistant may experience the same kinds of accelerated aging and tissue damage that occur in diabetics. Cardiovascular disease, high blood pressure, liver disease and kidney damage are just a few of the many complications that can arise from pre-diabetes.

What Is Metabolic Syndrome?

Metabolic syndrome, originally called Syndrome X by Stanford University endocrinologist Gerald Reaven, M.D., is a condition identified by a number of metabolic risk factors, including:

- central obesity (excessive fat tissue in and around the abdomen) shown by waist to hip ratio;
- low levels of HDL cholesterol (Less than 40 mg/dl for men and less than 50 mg/dl for women);
- fasting blood triglycerides greater than or equal to 150 mg/dl;
- elevated blood pressure (130/85 mmHg or higher); and
- insulin resistance (glucose levels between 101 and 125 mg/dl).

Metabolic syndrome is a serious health issue. People who have it are at increased risk for coronary artery disease, other diseases related to plaque buildup on the artery walls and Type 2 diabetes. The presence of four or more of the above criteria means you have more than double the risk of having a heart attack or stroke and nearly 25 times the risk of developing diabetes.

The Importance of Insulin

Insulin is an anabolic hormone that promotes the growth of both muscle and fat. But when insulin resistance develops, insulin continues to stimulate the growth of fat, but has little effect on muscle. As a result, the body tends to deposit fat and lose muscle mass. Because of this, it is very difficult for fat to be burned efficiently.

Insulin should act as the "off button" for appetite. But with insulin resistance, the appetite never really shuts down. In normal individuals, regions of the brain responsible for appetite regulation respond to after-meal elevations in insulin by significantly increasing their intake of glucose. This reaction causes a decrease in appetite and a sense of satiety. However, if you are insulin resistant this increase in metabolic activity is diminished, even after a significant rise in insulin levels. We now know that the brain becomes insulin resistant along with the rest of the body, and this insulin resistance prevents satiety and speeds weight gain.

Many people experience blood sugar surges after meals, followed by a rapid drop in blood sugar, creating weakness, agitation and shakiness.

Elevated Glycemic Volatility

Even if their blood sugar never drops below normal, many people experience blood sugar surges after meals, followed by a rapid drop in blood sugar. When blood sugar drops too quickly, adrenaline and cortisol are released, creating weakness, agitation and shakiness. Hunger pangs and brain fog can accompany a drop in blood sugar. The brain detects this rapidly dropping blood sugar and respond by sending out strong signals that it is time to eat. Commonly called hypoglycemia, rapidly fluctuating blood sugar levels are made worse by eating high glycemic foods.

Stop The Blood Sugar Roller Coaster

If you are riding the blood sugar roller coaster, it will be nearly impossible to lose weight. Frequent, rapid fluctuations in blood sugar can cause serious food cravings, even when your body has no real need for additional calories. If you succeed in resisting the cravings, your appetite will be in overdrive for the next meal and you could eat too much of the wrong foods. According to Drs. Murray and Lyon, there are five key steps to reducing blood sugar volatility and improving your ability to lose weight.

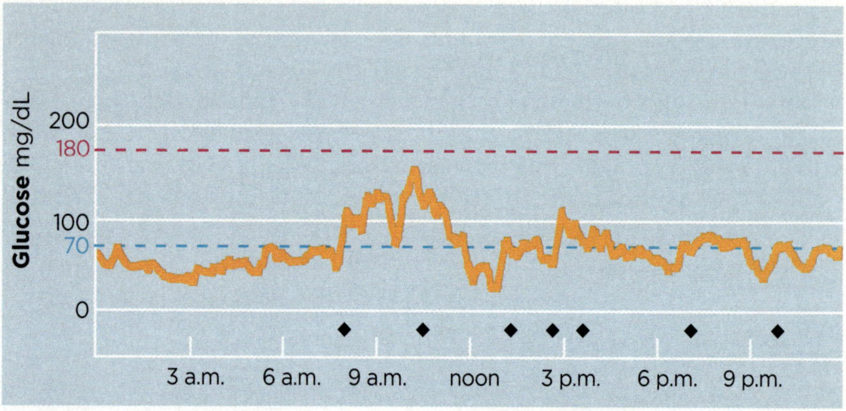

Figure 3.3 **In this case, black diamonds represent times when the patient feels "hypoglycemic" and then responds by eating. Each time represents an episode of rapidly dropping blood sugar, but only two occasions (while awake) are actual hypoglycemic episodes (below 70 mg/dl). Elevated glycemic volatility with rapid drops in blood sugar explains most "hypoglycemic" symptoms in non-diabetics. It is more commonly associated with food cravings or "hunger pangs."**

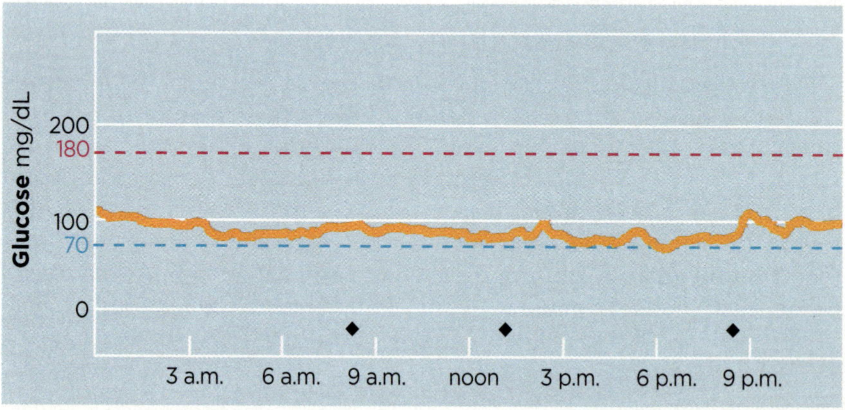

Figure 3.4 **Same patient after four weeks of using the PGX program. Hypoglycemic symptoms and excessive food cravings are resolved.**

1. Follow a low glycemic diet.
2. Increase your daily intake of dietary fiber and protein.
3. Take PGX with every meal.
4. Get regular exercise.
5. Take a high potency multiple vitamin with chromium daily.

The Glycemic Index and Glycemic Load

The glycemic index (GI) is a numerical scale used to indicate how fast and how high a particular food raises blood sugar levels. There are two versions of the GI. One compares foods using straight glucose as the control, giving it a value of 100. The other version compares foods to a slice of white bread. Refined sugars, white flour products and other sources of simple sugars are quickly absorbed into the bloodstream, causing a rapid rise in blood sugar. While you don't need to know the exact GI number of the foods you eat, it is very helpful to know if they are low, medium or high GI foods.

The GI is quite useful, but it doesn't tell you how much carbohydrate is in a typical serving of a particular food. That is where glycemic load (GL) comes in. GL is a way to assess the impact of carbohydrate consumption. A GL of 20 or more is high, a GL of 11 to 19 is medium and a GL of 10 or less is low. Foods, like beets, can have a high GI but low GL. Although the carbohydrates in beets have a high GI, a typical serving is small, so its GL is very low. If you eat a reasonable portion of a low GL food, the impact on blood sugar is acceptable, even if the food is high in its GI.

Table 3.3 **Samples of GI, GL And Glycemic Impact Scores of Selected Foods**

Food	GI	GL	Glycemic Impact
Carrots, cooked, 1/2 cup	49	1.5	low
Beets, cooked 1/2 cup	64	3	low
Whole wheat bread, 1 slice	69	9.6	low
Baked potato, medium	93	14	medium
Brown rice, cooked, 1 cup	50	16	medium
Banana, raw, 1 medium	55	17.6	medium
Spaghetti, white, cooked, 1 cup	41	23	high
White rice, cooked, 1 cup	72	26	high
Soft drinks, 375 ml (about 12.5 oz.)	68	34.7	very high

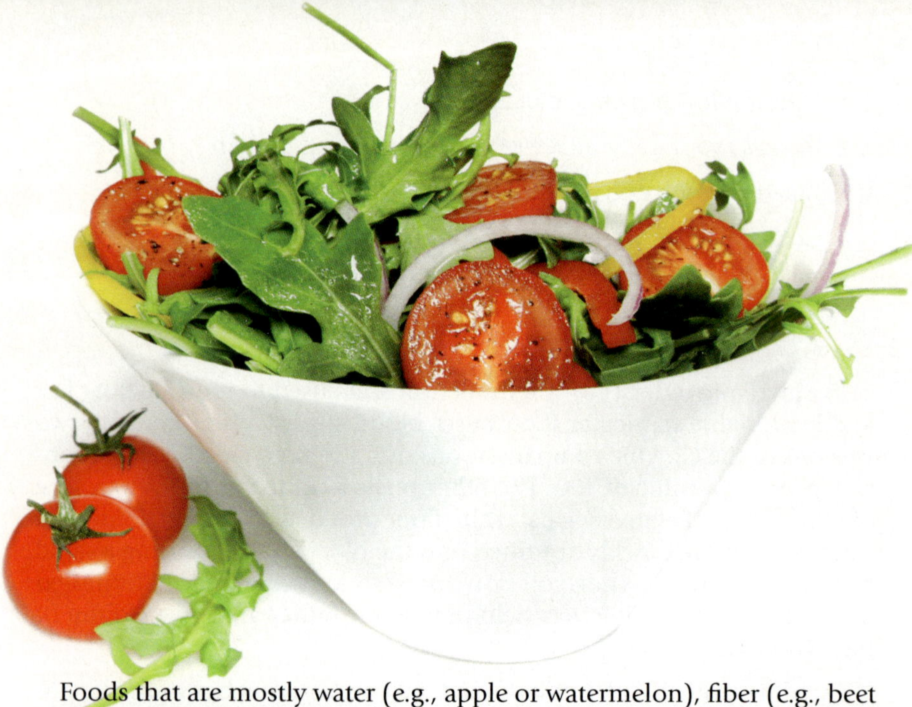

Foods that are mostly water (e.g., apple or watermelon), fiber (e.g., beet root or carrot) or air (e.g., popcorn) will not cause a steep rise in your blood sugar even if their GI is high as long as you keep portion sizes moderate. Try keeping your GL for any three hour period less than 20.

In a double-blind, placebo-controlled study presented at the American Diabetes Association, a three week program of PGX produced a 50 percent reduction in after-meal insulin levels and a 40 percent improvement in insulin sensitivity for participants, along with a significant decrease in after-meal blood sugars. Researchers found that when PGX was added to foods or beverages it greatly reduced its GI. This means that any food taken with PGX can have a substantially lower GI, and glycemic volatility (as shown in the previous graphs) is reduced within days of taking PGX.

PGX is easy to use, natural, colorless and has no distinctive odor or taste. Some fibers are non-thickening and cannot provide the health benefits of PGX. Other fiber products thicken too quickly and can make foods and beverages unpalatable. PGX in its granular form gels at a much slower rate, making it easy to mix into foods and beverages. PGX is also available in a convenient soft gel.

Research shows that adding PGX to a healthy diet and exercise program results in successful, sustainable weight loss. PGX can be found at most natural health stores throughout North America.

In addition to soluble fiber, there are other factors to consider if you want to lose weight.

Chapter Three

Other Important Factors

Let's face it for many people losing weight is not easy. That's because there are many factors that influence weight loss and weight gain. Even our sleep patterns can make us fat.

That's right, new research shows that lack of sleep can cause you to pack on the pounds. According to the International Journal of Obesity, individuals who are sleep-deprived have more body fat than those who sleep well. "These associations persisted after adjusting for sleep apnea, insomnia, and daytime sleepiness," concluded the researchers. In other words, even if you don't have a diagnosed sleep disorder you can still experience the damaging effects of sleep deprivation. The researchers also found that disrupted sleep cycles were associated with a higher body fat percentage, as well as a wider waistline.

This actually makes sense. While we sleep, chemicals and hormones that help control appetite are released. If we are not sleeping soundly, those chemical messengers and hormones are disrupted, which can cause us to gain weight. The take home message: If you want to lose weight, be sure to get between seven and nine hours of sleep every night.

Often, the reason we can't sleep is because we are experiencing a lot of stress. This creates a vicious cycle for those trying to lose weight because stress can also influence weight gain.

Stress Eating

We are faced with many stressors including issues with the economy, careers, family, health, and more. Even trying to lose weight is stressful because we know if we don't do it we are putting ourselves at risk of developing many serious illnesses.

Biologically, the human body has checks and balances that help us deal with stress. But when stress becomes chronic, it throws our system into constant survival mode. During times of stress, the body activates key hormones to help us cope. When elevated for an extended period of time, however, some of these hormones—specifically cortisol—do more harm than good. Our bodies are hardwired to stock up on fuel after stressful encounters. That means constantly high levels of cortisol actually increase our desire to eat. Worse yet, because our bodies use sugar as fuel, that's exactly what we crave. Suppressing appetite and controlling these stress-induced cravings becomes critical to weight loss.

Editor's Note: For more information about healthy ways to cope with stress, refer to the Better Nutrition Health Living Guide titled RELAX by Sherry Torkos, BSc, Phm, available at your local health store.

An effective stress-reducing technique is exercise. This is a perfect solution, because exercise is also a vital component to any long-lasting weight loss program.

Get Moving to Keep Losing

If you've read this far you know that there is a relationship between lean muscle, blood sugar and weight. Research shows exercise alone is of limited value as a weight loss strategy. In one of the latest studies in women, even substantial increases in exercise alone were not enough to produce weight loss. Reduced calorie intake was also needed. However men, largely due to an increase in muscle mass, were able to lose weight by simply increasing their exercise.

Muscle mass is the primary fat burning furnace of the body. The more muscle you have, the more fat you burn. A muscle cell burns as much as 15 times more calories per day than a fat cell. Muscle mass is also the primary factor in the speed of weight loss. Avoid radical diets that burn up muscle as they set you up for failure.

Moderate to intense exercise may also have an appetite suppressing effect that can help maintain a healthy weight. Plus, exercise helps to diminish anxiety and depression, two things that may cause over-eating. Lack of physical activity promotes insulin resistance while moderate exercise can help stabilize appetite, normalize blood sugar levels and increase muscle mass, improving your metabolic rate.

The Importance of Protein

Along with its satiety-promoting properties, dietary protein is essential for supporting muscle growth. You need adequate protein with every meal, including breakfast. Protein supplements can be used to balance out any meal that is low in protein or when you want a smoothie as a meal replacement. The best choice is whey protein. Even those who are lactose intolerant can usually use a high quality whey protein isolate or concentrate.

Whey protein has the highest biological value of all proteins. Biological value indicates how much of the protein consumed is actually absorbed,

Let's Get Physical

Being physically active on a consistent basis is one of the best ways to lose weight and keep it off. The most effective fitness program includes activities in cardiovascular endurance, involving the heart and lungs, muscular strength training and endurance, and flexibility. Walking, running, biking, hiking, and swimming are all examples of cardiovascular activities. Weight lifting and using resistance bands will help strengthen muscles, and yoga and stretching are ways to enhance flexibility.

Following are some general exercise tips:

- If you have been fairly sedentary for a long time, consult with your doctor before embarking on a vigorous exercise program.
- Find a fitness buddy to help keep you motivated.
- Drink plenty of water before, during, and after exercise.
- Mix it up and vary your routine so you don't become bored.
- Increase duration, frequency, and intensity as you are able.

The key to success is consistency and frequency. It is far better to exercise four times a week for 30 minutes rather than twice a week for one hour each time. Choose activities that you enjoy. If you prefer to be outside, work in the garden or go for a hike. If you are more social, exercise classes may be your fitness activity of choice.

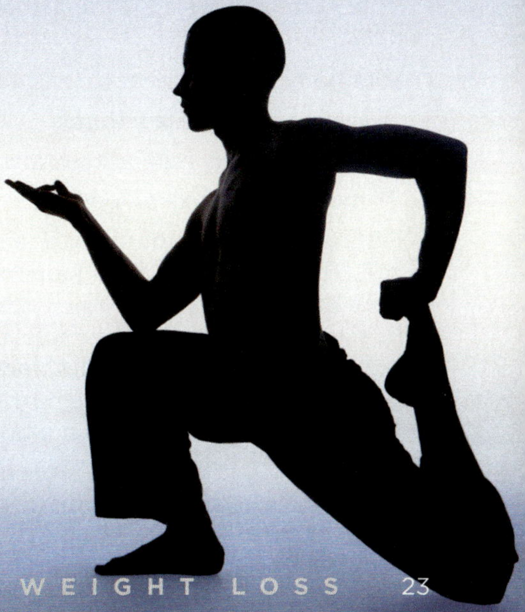

Moderate to intense exercise may also have an appetite suppressing effect that can help maintain a healthy weight.

retained and used by the body. It also provides amino acids that are critical to cellular health, muscle growth and protein synthesis. Although we most often think of whey protein as a supplement for body builders and athletes, it is an excellent protein source for anyone recovering from illness or surgery.

Retraining Your Metabolism

Have you ever had a friend who could eat all the food she wanted and still stay thin while simply looking at food goes right to your hips or belly? You have probably heard is that it is a difference in metabolism. But what exactly is metabolism and how does it relate to weight control?

Metabolism refers to the breakdown of food into the energy required for life. The amount of energy contained in any specific food is expressed in calories, which is simply a measurement of heat. Food is "burned" inside our cells and most of the energy is trapped to be used for thousands of bodily processes. Some energy is released as heat to keep our bodies warm.

If you consume more calories than your body can burn, excess calories will be stored as fat. In fact, even normal weight people store a great deal of energy. A lean, 155 pound man carries about 35 pounds of fat on his body, which stores about 150,000 calories of energy—theoretically enough to keep him alive for a couple of months of starvation. A 250 pound person with 50 percent body fat is carrying 125 pounds, or 437,500 calories, of energy as stored fat. This much fat could provide all of the energy required for almost one year!

Total Energy Expenditure

Your body consumes energy in three different ways:

- resting energy expenditure;
- activity energy expenditure; and
- the thermic effect of food.

Resting energy expenditure is the amount of energy your body consumes at rest. The brain, heart, liver, kidneys and muscles consume the majority of your daily calories even while you are sleeping. Exercise and other daily activities consume a more variable amount of calories, depending upon your occupation, your activities and your level of exercise. The thermic effect of food is the energy you burn digesting food, processing nutrients and generating heat to warm your body.

Most overweight or obese people do not suffer from a low resting metabolic rate. In fact, as you gain weight, you are gaining mostly fat, but also some muscle. Muscle burns more energy at rest than fat, but even fat at rest burns some calories. Studies show that resting metabolic rate increases as body weight increases. Most overweight and obese people have high resting metabolic rates.

The best way to increase your resting metabolic rate is through a regular program of strength training. If you increase lean muscle mass, you will burn more calories around the clock. Improving insulin sensitivity can also help preserve your resting metabolism.

Thyroid: Master Gland of Metabolism

Before any further discussion of metabolism, be sure to find out from your doctor if your thyroid gland is functioning properly. This small gland in your neck secretes two hormones that regulate metabolism. Low levels of these thyroid hormones, called hypothyroidism, affects one in five women and a smaller percentage of men. If your thyroid activity is not optimum, your metabolism can be significantly impaired and you will have a tough time losing weight.

Thyroid hormones affect every cell of the body. A deficiency can cause symptoms like low body temperature, intolerance to cold, weight gain or an inability to lose weight, depression, lack of concentration, hair loss and fatigue. If you have any of these symptoms, check with your doctor to determine if you have an under-active thyroid. Medical treatment of hypothyroidism usually involves the use of natural or synthetic thyroid hormones. However, be aware that taking prescription thyroid hormones will not promote weight loss and is actually linked to loss of muscle mass and bone.

Support Liver Health

The liver is involved in all aspects of metabolism and plays a central role in processing fat, protein and carbohydrates. Many overweight individuals develop what is known as a fatty liver, a condition that can interfere with metabolism.

The best ways to support your liver are to avoid putting too much stress on it and giving it the nutritional building blocks it needs to function properly. Don't smoke. Drink little or no alcohol. Avoid drugs that can harm the liver—even acetaminophen—and avoid harmful chemicals, especially cleaning solvents and pesticides.

In general, supporting your liver involves the same actions and preventive steps needed to support good general health: Avoid trans fats, deep fried foods, refined sugar and alcohol, drink at least 48 ounces of water each day, and consume plenty of vegetables and legumes for their high fiber and nutrient content.

Chapter Four

Build A Satisfying Relationship With Food

Most foods in the modern Western diet are packed with calories relative to the amount of volume they occupy in the stomach. This can make you eat many more calories than you need before your stomach feels full. For example, a double burger with cheese and a large order of fries occupies about two cups of volume in your stomach, but contributes about 1,300 calories. Since the stomach of an obese person can hold up to four quarts of volume, the two cups of burger and fries wouldn't necessarily create a sense of fullness even though the calorie intake is huge. On the other hand, two cups of chopped apple gives you only 120 calories. You would have to eat 22 cups of chopped apple to consume the same number of calories as that burger and those fries!

Viscosity is Vital

Typical foods in the Western diet are very low in viscosity. They become a thin watery liquid once they are chewed, swallowed and mixed with fluids and acid in the stomach. Low viscosity foods move through the digestive tract quickly and are rapidly absorbed, leaving your body looking

Want to Get REALLY FAT, REALLY FAST?

These are the foods that will take you there, so avoid them at all cost!

- Ice cream
- Cookies, cakes and pies
- Donuts and pastries
- White bread and white flour products
- Fried foods, especially deep fried
- White sugar, chocolate and candy
- Pop, fruit juice and other sugary drinks
- Bacon, sausage, wieners and processed meats
- Hot dogs and fast food burgers
- Potato chips and tortilla chips
- White rice
- Sugary breakfast cereals

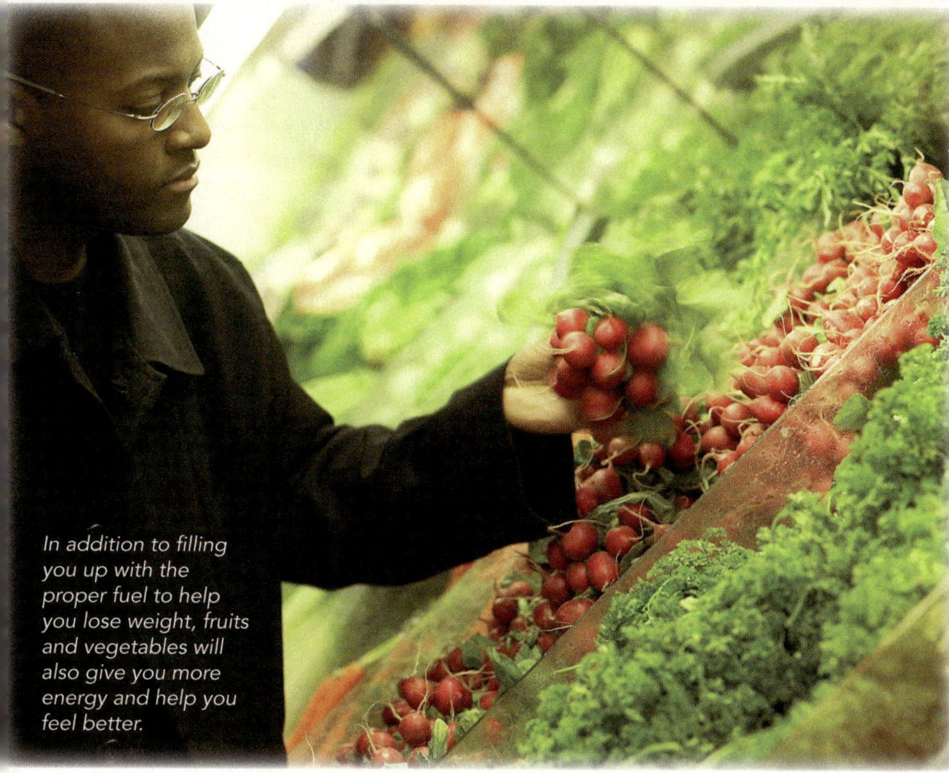

In addition to filling you up with the proper fuel to help you lose weight, fruits and vegetables will also give you more energy and help you feel better.

for more food shortly after you've eaten. Foods containing highly refined carbohydrates cause a rapid and excessive rise in blood sugar. They can provide fast satisfaction, but it doesn't last.

To promote satiety, you need a variety of foods each day that are low in calories, high in volume and viscosity, yet low in glycemic impact. For example, if you take two PGX capsules daily one-half hour before a meal and start with a large salad or high-fiber soup, you will start to feel full before the entrée. This gives your stomach a chance to communicate to the brain that you are satisfied before you turn to the higher calorie foods in your meal.

The Science of Satiety

PGX absorbs several hundred times its weight in water, adding to the volume of your meal without adding calories. When mixed with water, it becomes the most viscous dietary fiber ever developed. PGX mixes with food, increasing its viscosity, slowing gastric emptying and prolonging the digestion and absorption of any food. It also slows the absorption of carbohydrates, lowering the glycemic impact of these foods. Eating less and feeling satisfied can help contribute to successful weight loss.

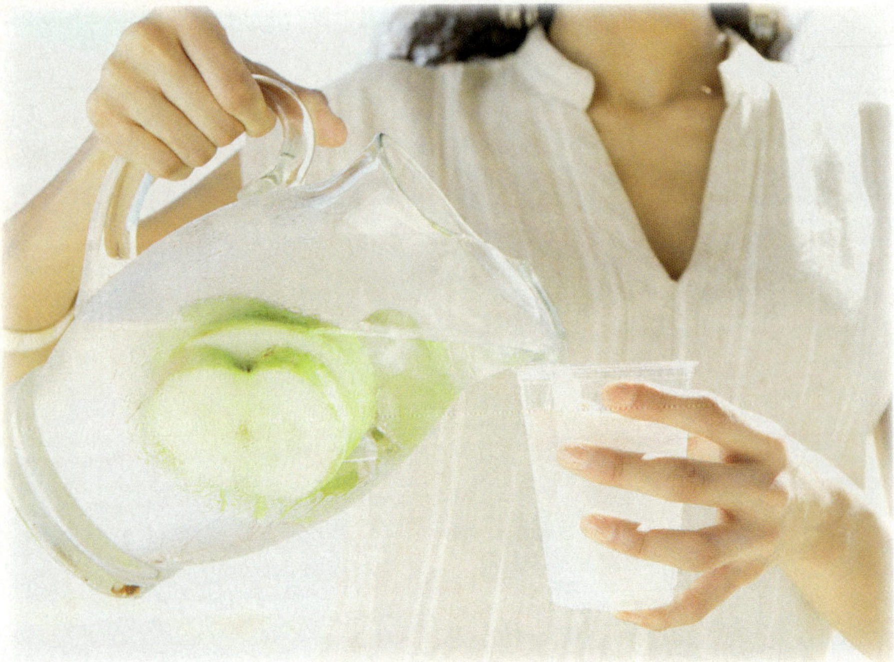

Additional Dietary Considerations

Fiber And Caloric Density

Fiber and water are the two most important ingredients in food for adding volume and viscosity without contributing calories. Fiber refers to carbohydrates that cannot be digested. They contribute very few calories. Fiber can be insoluble (it doesn't absorb much water) or soluble. High fiber foods help you to feel full on fewer calories. Here are a few satiety stars:

- low-fat salads;
- high-fiber soups;
- beans and legumes;
- raw or cooked non-starchy vegetables;
- boiled whole grains like brown rice or oatmeal; and
- low fat stews.

In addition to consuming high satiety foods, you can add PGX to your meals two to three times per day. A dosage of 2.5 to 5 grams of PGX powder or granules can be taken before meals or added to soups, yogurt or any moist food. PGX is also available in capsules and in PGX Daily softgels, as well as delicious meal replacement beverage mixes. PGX acts quickly in the stomach to create a sense of fullness, slow digestion and promote healthy blood sugar levels already within normal range, making weight loss much easier.

Cool, Clear Water

Maybe you're not hungry - maybe you're thirsty. In many cases, a hunger pang can be relieved by simply drinking a glass of water. Mild dehydration creates a sensation that is similar to hunger. Those who successfully lose weight and keep it off have learned to drink plenty of water. They also eat low-fat, high-fiber soups, vegetables, fruits, boiled whole grains and other volumetric foods. The fiber in these foods holds on to the water and increases their volume.

Plant-Based Diet is Best

One of the healthiest ways to achieve your weight loss goals is to stick with a plant-based diet. This type of diet focuses more on colorful fruits and vegetables. Here are the key components of a weight loss plant-based diet:

- eat more fish and less red meat
- eat healthy oils such as olive, avocado, and macadamia nut in place of butter and margarine
- eat at least five servings of fruits and vegetables every day
- eat more nuts and seeds

In addition to filling you up with the proper fuel to help you lose weight, these foods will also give you more energy and help you feel better.

Knowing When You Have Had Enough

The body really doesn't know how many calories you've consumed until the food is digested and fully absorbed. This is why it is so easy to overeat. You can easily eat 2,000 calories of fast food in a few minutes and not even realize that you've eaten three times your caloric requirements for that meal until some time later when you feel very full. Research shows that most people with weight problems eat faster and swallow more food within the same time period as people of normal weight. That is why one of the simplest and most effective strategies for losing weight is to eat more slowly, savoring every bite.

Your mother probably warned you not to "spoil your appetite" by eating between meals. In reality, your worst enemy is excessive hunger. You will lose weight more easily if you don't allow yourself to get really hungry. Instead, spread your calories throughout the day. A handful of carrots, a hard-boiled egg or a couple pieces of celery can be eaten one-half to one hour before dinner to reduce hunger and prevent overeating. Adding 2.5 to 5 grams of PGX to a glass of water and drinking it 15 to 20 minutes before each meal will make a major change in your appetite.

Protein, Fat, And Satiety

Both fat and protein contribute to a food's taste as well its ability to initiate and maintain satiety. Even though fat is high in calories, you need some healthy fats if you want to lose weight. The biggest mistake is eating too much fat, and thus too many calories. As little as two grams of fat in a stomach full of food can vastly increase satiety. The essential fatty acids in olive oil, avocado, nuts and seeds, fatty fish, fish oils and coconut oil should be consumed regularly for health and satiety. All fats contain about nine calories per gram so moderation is the key.

Cell membranes are made mostly of fatty acids. Saturated fats and trans fatty acids (from margarine, shortening and other sources of hydrogenated vegetable oils) make membranes that are much less fluid than the membranes in a person who consumes optimum levels of unsaturated fatty acids. Without a healthy membrane, cells lose their ability to hold water and nutrients. They also lose their ability to communicate with other cells and to be controlled by regulating hormones, including insulin. Cell membrane dysfunction is a critical factor in the development of insulin resistance, obesity and diabetes. To improve insulin action, reduce your intake of saturated fats and eliminate trans fatty acids.

The right oils are omega-3-rich fish oils from salmon, mackerel, herring or halibut. Add a high quality fish oil supplement to your diet to get the benefits of eating fish without the concerns about mercury, PCBs, dioxins and other contaminants. Be sure to get 1,000 mg daily of the key omega-3 fatty acids, EPA and DHA. I recommend Dr. Murray's RX Omega-3 Factors.

Eating protein throughout the day also helps improve appetite control. It is particularly important to start the day with a high-protein breakfast. Eggs or egg whites with grilled vegetables, grilled chicken with vegetables, yogurt and bran cereal, scrambled tofu with vegetables, or a high protein meal replacement drink or smoothie with PGX are excellent for satiety support.

One of the best sources of protein for weight loss is legumes which also contain soluble fiber. Learn to cook a variety of beans, lentils, split peas and other legume products such as tofu. What about cheese? While it is true that cheese is high in protein, it is also high in calories. Keep portions small, about the size of your thumb.

Final Thoughts

Diets don't work. In fact, they can cause you to feel frustrated and hungry. The key to long-lasting weight loss is appetite and blood sugar control. When you control your appetite and feel satisfied, you can shift your thinking and change your relationship with food. This is not a diet, it's a new way of living.

To make this important shift, there are key changes you must make in your diet and lifestyle. The first is to increase your consumption of soluble fiber. As mentioned previously, I highly recommend PGX because it is the most viscous dietary fiber ever developed. In addition to PGX, increase your consumption of fruits and vegetables, water, and healthy proteins. Take control of your response to stress, get plenty of sleep, and exercise consistently. This plan will not only help you lose weight, it will help you keep it off. Remember, when you maintain your weight loss, you also help prevent some of the most serious illnesses in North America including cancer, heart disease, and diabetes. You will also feel better and have the energy you need to live life with vitality.

Selected References

Behall KM, Scholdfield DJ, Lee K, et al. Mineral balance in adult men: effects of four refined fibers. *American Journal of Clinical Nutrition* 46(2): 307-314, 1987.

Behall KM, Scholfield DJ, McIvor ME, et al. Effect of guar gum on mineral balances in NIDDM adults. *Diabetes Care* 12 (5): 357-364, 1989.

Behall KM. Effects of soluble fibers on plasma, glucose tolerance and mineral balance. *Advances in Experimental Medicine and Biology* 270: 7-16, 1990.

Breitman P, Vuksan V, Lyon, M. Impact of meal replacement viscosity on appetite and ad-libitum food consumption in normal weight adolescents. Presented at the 8th Annual Canadian Diabetes Association (CDA)/Canadian Society of Endocrinology and Metabolism (CSEM) Professional Conference, Quebec City, October, 2004.

Coudray C, Bellanger J, Castiglia-Delavaud C, et al. Effects of soluble or partly soluble dietary fibers supplementation on absorption and balance of calcium, magnesium, iron and zinc in healthy young men. *European Journal of Clinical Nutrition* 51(6): 375-80, 1997.

Glycemic Index Laboratories. Report: Determination of glycemic index lowering potential of PGX in liquid and solid food formulations. August 2, 2006.

Greger JL. Nondigestible carbohydrates and mineral bioavailability. J Nutr 129 (7 Suppl):1434S-5S, 1999.

Griffin IJ, Davila PM, Abrams SA. Non-digestible oligosaccharides and calcium absorption in girls with adequate calcium intakes. *British Journal of Nutrition* 87 Suppl 2: S187-191, 2002.

Jenkins AL, Panahi S, Azatagagha A, et al. Effects of different fibers on bowel habits in healthy individuals. Presented at FASEB, Washington D.C. 2006.

Jenkins AL, Morgan L, Zdravkovic U, et al. Importance of administration mode of viscous fiber (VF) on postprandial glycemia. Presented at the 8th Annual Canadian Diabetes Association (CDA)/Canadian Society of Endocrinology and Metabolism (CSEM) Professional Conference, Quebec City, poster #93 October 2004.

Jenkins DJ, Wolever TM, Leeds AR, et al. Dietary fibers, fiber analogues and glucose tolerance: importance of viscosity. *British Medical Journal* 1:1392-1394, 1978.

Livieri C, Novazi F, Lorini R. Usefulness of highly purified glucomannan fibers in childhood obesity. *La Pediatria medica e chirurgica : Medical and surgical pediatrics* 14:195-198, 1992.

Ministry of Industry, 2006. Statistics Canada Catalogue No. 21-020-XIE. *Food Statistics* 5 (1), 2005.

Patel SR, et al. The association between sleep duration and obesity in older adults. *Int J Obes*, Oct 21, 2008.

Rogovik A, Jenkins AL, Breitman P, et al. A blend of highly viscous polysaccharides decreases relative CVD risk in three population groups. Natural Health Product Research Conference, Toronto 2006.

Tahari M, Tressol JC, Arnaud J, et al. Five-week intake of short-chain fructo-oligosaccharides increases intestinal absorption and status of magnesium in postmenopausal women. *Journal of Bone and Mineral Research* 16(11): 2152-2160, 2001.

United States Department of Health and Human Services and U.S. Department of Agriculture. Dietary Guidelines for Americans 2005. 6th edition, Washington DC: U.S. Government Printing Office, January 2005

Vuksan V, Sievenpiper JL, Owen R, et al. Beneficial effects of viscous dietary fiber from Konjac-mannan in subjects with the insulin resistance syndrome: results of a controlled metabolic trial. *Diabetes Care* 23 (1): 9-14, 2000.

Vuksan V, Lyon M, Breitman P et al. 3-Week Consumption of a Highly Viscous dietary fiber blend results in improvements in insulin sensitivity and reductions in body fat: Results of a double blind, placebo controlled trial. Presented at the 64th Annual Meeting of the American Diabetes Association. Orlando, Florida; June 4-8, 2004

Vuksan V, Jenkins DJ, Spadafora P, et al. Konjac-mannan (glucomannan) improves glycemia and other associated risk factors for coronary heart disease in Type 2 diabetes. A randomized controlled metabolic trial. *Diabetes Care* 22 (6): 913-919, 1999.

Yun-Hua H, Li-Shi Z, Hong-Ming Z, et al. Influences of refined konjac meal on the levels of tissue lipids and the absorption of four minerals in rats. *Biomedical and Environmental Science* 3: 306-314, 1990.

Zhang MY, Peng SS, Zhang YZ, et al. Long-term animal feeding trial of the refined konjac meal. I. Effects of the refined konjac meal on the calcium and phosphours metabolism and the bone in rats. *Biomedical and Environmental Science* 8(1): 74-79, 1995.

www.pgx.com

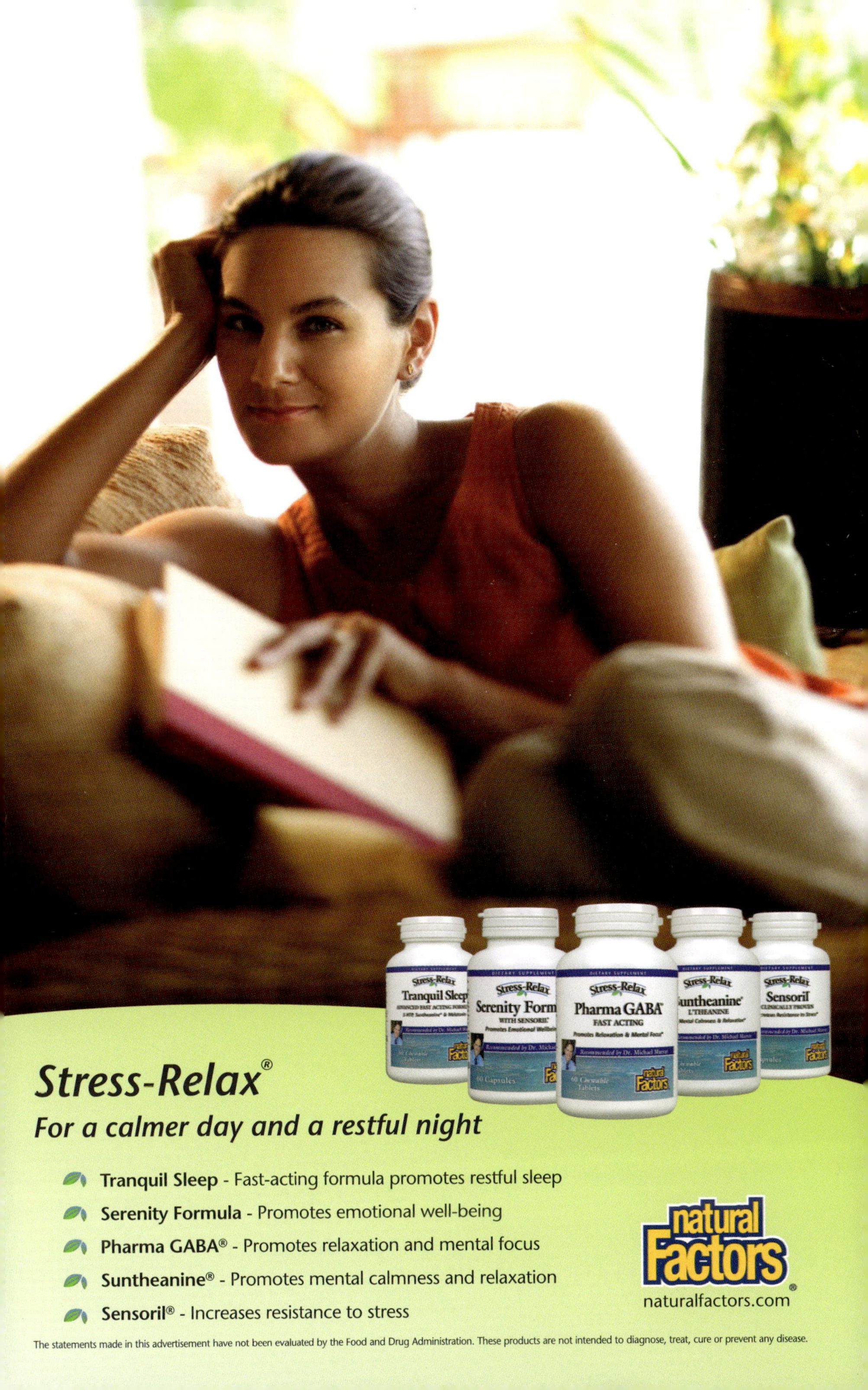
Stress-Relax®
For a calmer day and a restful night
Tranquil Sleep - Fast-acting formula promotes restful sleep
Serenity Formula - Promotes emotional well-being
Pharma GABA® - Promotes relaxation and mental focus
Suntheanine® - Promotes mental calmness and relaxation
Sensoril® - Increases resistance to stress
natural Factors®
naturalfactors.com
The statements made in this advertisement have not been evaluated by the Food and Drug Administration. These products are not intended to diagnose, treat, cure or prevent any disease.

WEIGHT LOSS

ALL-NATURAL **APPETITE CONTROL** AND **BLOOD SUGAR BALANCE**

There are two key barriers to weight loss: Increased appetite and insulin sensitivity. In this booklet, naturopathic doctor Kate Rhéaume-Bleue explains how an innovative new fiber substance can help break down those two barriers. Dr. Rhéaume-Bleue provides detailed information about the scientific studies associated with this substance. She includes testimonials from the research participants and provides readers with an overview of why and how this substance works. She also gives readers advice about an effective weight loss diet and lifestyle.

ABOUT THE AUTHOR OF THIS BOOKLET

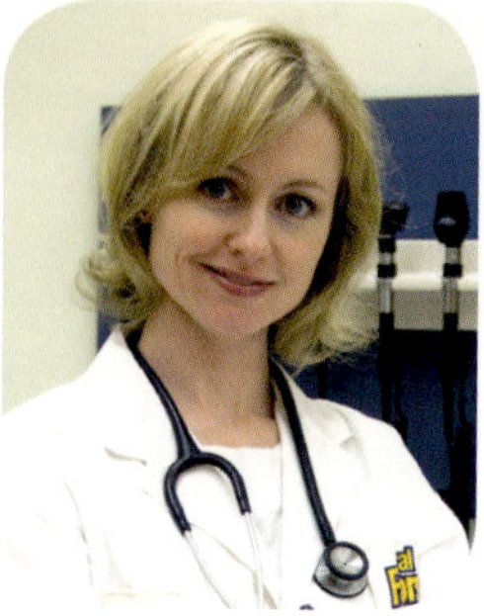

Kate Rhéaume-Bleue, ND, is a doctor of naturopathic medicine, writer and educator. A former faculty member at the Canadian College of Naturopathic Medicine, Dr. Rhéaume-Bleue is a Canadian expert in the field of natural health and speaks across the country on topics related to natural medicine. She is also a contributing editor to several health-related publications.

ISBN 978-1-935297-20-8

50495

9 781935 297208

better nutrition healthy living guide

betternutrition.com